EATING HEALTHY WITH DR. FRANCIS

101 Quick & Easy

30 MINUTE RECIPES

-for-

DIABETICS

Dr. A. Francis

December | 2022

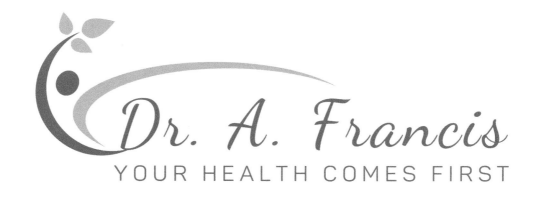

YOUR HEALTH COMES FIRST

Copyright © 2022 T.C.PASK

All rights reserved

ISBN 979-8-9873520-1-4

t.c.paskpublishing@gmail.com

LUNCHES

DINNERS

BONUS RECIPES

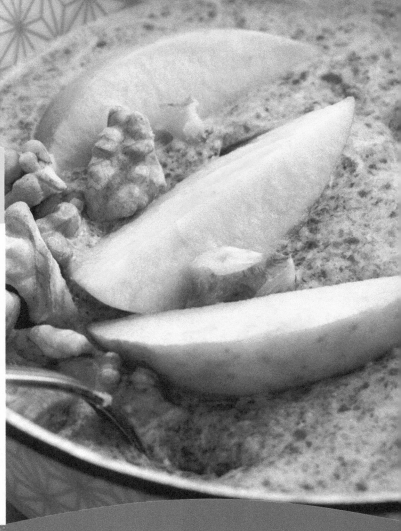

BREAKFASTS

AIR FRYER MEALS

ASIAN LETTUCE *Wraps*

Lunch

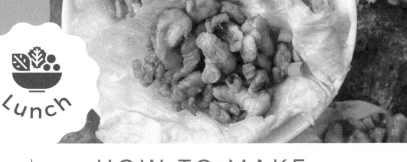

INGREDIENTS
For 4 servings

- 1 lb cooked chicken breast, *shredded*
- 1 cup shredded cabbage
- Large lettuce leaves
- 2 scallions, *thinly sliced*
- 6 tsp peanut sauce

HOW TO MAKE

- Spoon chicken, cabbage into lettuce leaves. Add scallions.
- Drizzle with peanut sauce.

TURKEY & CHICKPEA *Stew*

Dinner

INGREDIENTS
For 4 servings

- 1 tbsp olive oil
- 1 lb lean ground turkey
- 2 cans chickpeas, *drained*
- 1 medium onion, *chopped*
- 2 medium carrots, *diced*
- 4 cloves garlic, *minced*
- 3 tbsp tomato paste
- 4 cups chicken broth
- 3 cups spinach

HOW TO MAKE

- Mash 1 can chickpeas.
- Heat oil in a large pot over medium-high heat. Add turkey, onion, carrots, garlic, cook 3 mins.
- Add tomato paste, broth, salt, mashed and whole chickpeas.
- Cover and bring to a simmer (about 10 mins).
- Add spinach, cook 2 mins.

VEG HUMMUS
Sandwiches

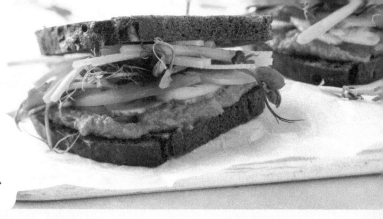

Lunch

INGREDIENTS

For 4 servings

- 1 cup cucumber, *sliced*
- 8 slices whole-grain bread
- 1 medium bell pepper, *sliced*
- 2 cups mixed salad greens
- 12 tbsp beetroot hummus
- 1 cup carrot, *shredded*
- 1 avocado, *mashed*

HOW TO MAKE

- Spread one slice of bread with avocado, the other with hummus. Top with veggies.
- Slice in half and serve.

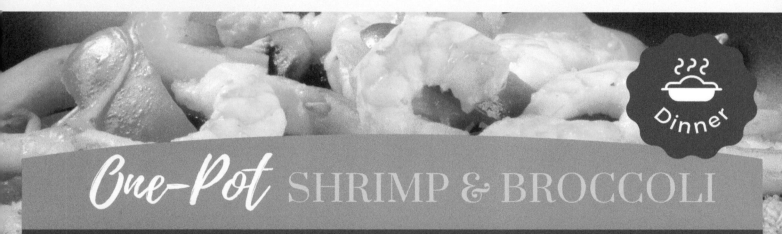

Dinner

One-Pot SHRIMP & BROCCOLI

INGREDIENTS

For 4 servings

- 1 lb shrimp, *peeled*
- 4 cups broccoli florets
- ½ cup bell pepper, *diced*
- 6 cloves garlic, *sliced*
- 2 tsp lemon juice
- 3 tbsp olive oil

HOW TO MAKE

- Heat 2 tbsp oil in a saucepan over medium heat. Add garlic, cook about 1 min. Add bell pepper, broccoli, salt, pepper. Cover and cook 5 mins. Transfer to a bowl.
- Add 1 tbsp oil to the pot. Add shrimp, cook 5 mins. Return the broccoli mixture to the pot, add lemon juice and stir to combine.

CHICKPEA *Wraps*

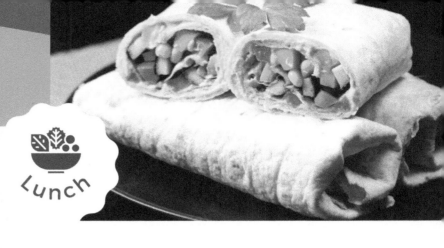

Lunch

INGREDIENTS

For 4 servings

- 1 tsp sugar free hot sauce
- 2 cans chickpeas, *drained*
- ½ cup cucumber sticks
- 2 cups romaine lettuce
- 1 cup carrot, *shredded*
- 4 whole-wheat wraps
- ¾ cup greek yogurt

HOW TO MAKE

- Roast the chickpeas 20 mins.
- Combine yogurt and hot sauce.
- Divide all ingredients among wraps. Roll up. Cut in half.

Dinner

SWEET POTATO *Enchiladas*

INGREDIENTS

For 4 servings

- ¾ cup pinto beans, *rinsed*
- 1 cup yellow onion, *sliced*
- ½ cup low carb enchilada sauce
- 3 tbsp reduced-fat cheese
- 1 sweet potato, *peeled and cut into cubes*
- 1 tbsp olive oil
- 12 egg wraps

HOW TO MAKE

- Microwave sweet potato with water about 5 mins. Drain.
- Heat oil in a medium skillet. Add onion, beans, sweet potato, cook 2 mins. Stir in sauce.
- Spoon 3 tbsp of potato mixture into egg wrap. Fold the wrap. Repeat with all wraps.
- Broil 3 mins. Sprinkle cheese over wraps.

VEGGIE PASTA *Salad*

Lunch

INGREDIENTS
For 4 servings

- 6 oz whole-wheat pasta
- 8 oz cherry tomatoes, halved
- ¾ cup reduced-fat feta cheese
- 1 medium zucchini, *chopped*
- 1 cup broccoli, *chopped*
- 2 tsp olive oil

HOW TO MAKE

- Heat oil in skillet. Add broccoli, zucchini, tomatoes. Cook 5 mins.
- Cook pasta. Mix vegetables with pasta. Toss in feta cheese.

Dinner

TERIYAKI CHICKEN *Quinoa Bowl*

INGREDIENTS
For 4 servings

- 2 cups cooked quinoa
- 2 medium chicken breasts
- 4 tbsp apple cider vinegar
- 3 tsp Monk fruit sweetener
- 4 tbsp coconut aminos
- 1 cup green beans
- 1 tsp garlic powder
- 2 tsp ground ginger
- 4 tsp almond flour

HOW TO MAKE

- Preheat 1 tbsp oil in a skillet. Add chicken. Cook 10 mins.
- Whisk together coconut aminos, sweetener, ginger, garlic powder, almond flour, vinegar to make sauce.
- Add green beans to chicken. Pour sauce and simmer until chicken is fully cooked.
- Serve with cooked quinoa.

TUNA SALAD *Wraps*

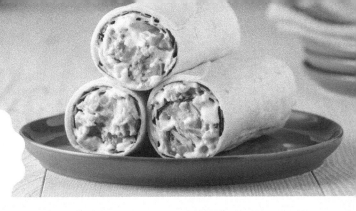

Lunch

INGREDIENTS
For 4 servings

- 1 stalk celery, *diced*
- 4 whole-wheat wraps
- 4 cans (4 oz) tuna, *drained*
- 1 cup greek yogurt
- 1 red bell pepper
- 1 cup spinach

HOW TO MAKE

- Drain tuna. Add yogurt, bell pepper, celery to the tuna. Mix.
- Divide mixture, spinach among wraps. Roll up. Cut in half.

ALASKA HALIBUT *with Quinoa*

Dinner

INGREDIENTS
For 4 servings

- 3 tbsp olive oil
- 2 tbsp lemon juice
- 1 tbsp parsley, *minced*
- 1 tsp garlic, *minced*
- ¼ tsp black pepper
- 4 four-ounce halibut fillets
- 2 cups quinoa
- ¼ cup spinach

HOW TO MAKE

- Preheat oven to 400°F.
- In a baking dish, add halibut skin side down, drizzle with oil.
- Top with parsley, garlic, lemon juice. Season with salt and pepper.
- Bake for 15 mins. Drizzle with lemon juice, serve with cooked quinoa and spinach.

SHRIMP & BEAN *Salad*

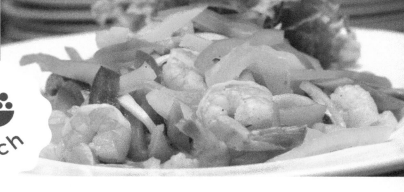

INGREDIENTS

For 4 servings

Lunch

- 1 lb cooked shrimp
- 1 can (15 oz) black beans
- 1 red bell pepper, *chopped*
- 1 cucumber, chopped
- ½ cup fresh cilantro
- 2 tbsp olive oil
- 1 tbsp fresh lime juice

HOW TO MAKE

- In a large bowl combine all ingredients, add salt to taste, mix well, toss until the shrimp are well coated.

Dinner

Tilapia AND ZUCCHINI NOODLES

INGREDIENTS

For 4 servings

- 2 large zucchini
- ½ tsp ground cumin
- ½ tsp smoked paprika
- 4 tilapia fillets (6 oz each)
- 2 garlic cloves, minced
- ¼ tsp garlic powder
- 1 cup pico de gallo
- ½ tsp pepper
- 2 tsp olive oil

HOW TO MAKE

- Using a spiralizer, cut zucchini into thin strands.
- Mix all spices and salt to taste, sprinkle onto tilapia.
- In a large skillet, heat oil over medium-high heat. Cook tilapia until fish begins to flake easily with a fork. Remove from skillet.
- Cook zucchini with garlic, about 2 mins. Serve with pico de gallo.

CHICKEN & EGG *Salad*

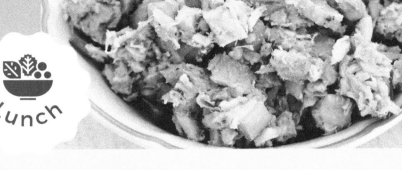

Lunch

INGREDIENTS
For 4 servings

- 4 chicken breasts
- 2 tbsp fat-free mayo
- 1 tbsp curry powder
- 4 hard-boiled eggs
- 1 cup avocado, *cubes*

HOW TO MAKE

- Bake chicken at 365°F for 20 mins.
- Cut chicken and eggs. Combine everything in a bowl, add salt to taste.

Dinner

TURKEY CABBAGE *Stew*

INGREDIENTS
For 4 servings

- 1 lb ground turkey
- 1 can diced tomatoes
- 1 medium onion, *chopped*
- 3 garlic cloves, *minced*
- 3 cups cabbage, *chopped*
- 2 medium carrots, *sliced*
- 1 tsp dried oregano
- ¼ tsp dried thyme
- ¾ cup water

HOW TO MAKE

- Cook the turkey, onion, and garlic in a large saucepan over medium heat until meat is no longer pink.
- Stir in remaining ingredients.
- Let simmer 10 mins (until vegetables are tender).

TUNA NICOISE *Salad*

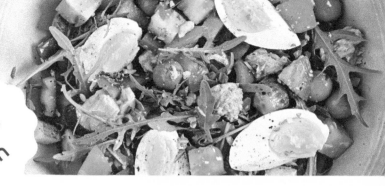

Lunch

INGREDIENTS

For 4 servings

- 1½ cup arugula
- ⅓ cup light Italian salad dressing
- 4 boiled eggs, *quartered*
- ¼ cup olives
- 1 can (10 oz) tuna, *drained*
- 2 cups grape tomatoes

HOW TO MAKE

- In a large bowl, add arugula and dressing, toss well to combine.
- Arrange on a platter. Top with the eggs, olives, tuna, tomatoes.

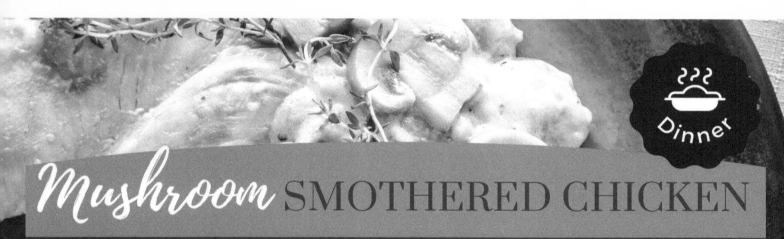

Dinner

Mushroom SMOTHERED CHICKEN

INGREDIENTS

For 4 servings

- 1 tsp olive oil
- ¾ cups sliced mushrooms
- 3 green onions, sliced
- 2 cups fresh baby spinach
- 4 tbsp chopped pecans
- 4 chicken breast halves
- 2 slices reduced-fat provolone cheese, *halved*

HOW TO MAKE

- In a large skillet, heat oil, saute mushrooms and green onions until tender. Stir in spinach and pecans until spinach is wilted. Remove from heat.
- Preheat oven to 425°F. Sprinkle chicken with salt. Bake for 20 mins.
- Top with cheese and mushroom mixture.

EASY SALMON *Wraps*

Lunch

INGREDIENTS
For 4 servings

- 8 oz. smoked salmon
- 8 tsp low fat cream cheese
- ½ cup red onion, *thinly sliced*
- 4 8-inch whole grain tortillas
- 2 tsp fresh or dried basil
- 1 cup arugula

HOW TO MAKE

- Warm tortillas in the oven.
- Mix together the cream cheese, basil, spread it onto the tortillas.
- Top it off with salmon, onion, arugula. Roll up and serve.

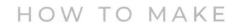

Dinner

ASPARAGUS & TURKEY *Stir-Fry*

INGREDIENTS
For 4 servings

- 1 lb ground turkey
- 1 lb frozen cut asparagus
- 1 cup carrots, *shredded*
- 4 green onions, *sliced*
- 2 cloves garlic, *minced*
- ¼ cup coconut aminos
- ¼ cup sweet chilli sauce, *sugar free*
- ¼ cup fresh basil, *sliced*

HOW TO MAKE

- Cook ground turkey in a large skillet over medium heat, until turkey is browned.
- Stir in carrots, garlic, green onions, asparagus, cook 2 mins.
- Stir in chili sauce, basil and coconut aminos, cook 3 mins.

Savory OATMEAL

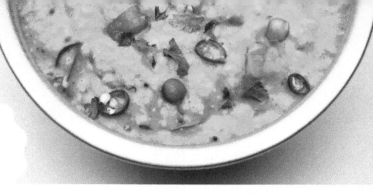

Lunch

INGREDIENTS
For 4 servings

- 4 cups vegetable broth
- 12 large sun-dried tomato
- 12 tbsp fat-free greek yogurt
- 4 tsp fresh cilantro, *sliced*
- 4 tbsp goat cheese, *crumbled*
- ¼ tsp turmeric powder
- 2 cups rolled oats

HOW TO MAKE

- Bring the broth, tomatoes to boil.
- Stir in the oats, reduce heat to medium. Cook 5 mins, stirring. Stir in yogurt. Serve with cilantro and cheese.

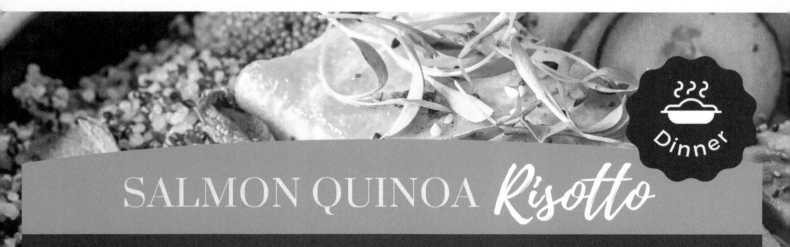

Dinner

SALMON QUINOA *Risotto*

INGREDIENTS
For 4 servings

- 1 medium yellow onion, *diced*
- 2 cups vegetable broth
- 4 cups almond milk
- 4 tsp italian herbs
- 4 salmon fillets
- 2 cups cooked quinoa
- 2 tsp olive oil

HOW TO MAKE

- Heat up olive oil in a skillet. Add onion, sauté for 2 mins.
- Add quinoa, almond milk, vegetable broth and Italian herbs. Cook 20 mins, stirring.
- Heat up a skillet. Add salmon fillets, let sear for 3 mins on each side. Season with salt.
- Serve salmon with quinoa and your favorite vegetables.

TUNA CHICKPEA *Pita*

Lunch

INGREDIENTS
For 4 servings

- 2 whole wheat pita
- 2 cans (10 oz) tuna, *drained*
- ½ cup *fat-free* greek yogurt
- 1 can (15 oz) chickpeas, *drained*
- ¼ cup fresh parsley
- 2 tbsp lemon juice
- 1 cup lettuce

HOW TO MAKE

- To a medium mixing bowl, add tuna, chickpeas, lettuce. Pour the greek yogurt, lemon juice, parsley.
- Slice pita pockets in half. Add tuna salad mixture.

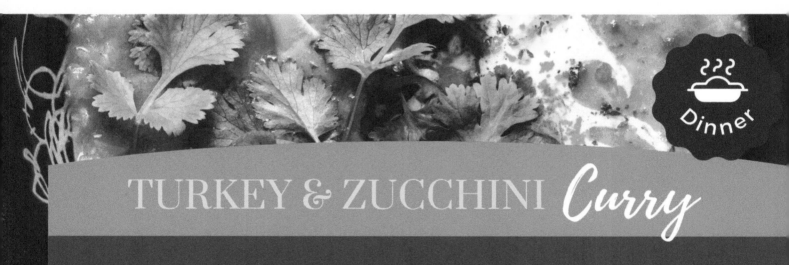

Dinner

TURKEY & ZUCCHINI *Curry*

INGREDIENTS
For 4 servings

- 2 tbsp olive oil
- 2 shallots, *thinly sliced*
- 1 cup zucchini, *chopped*
- 1 tbsp ginger, *minced*
- 1½ tbsp curry powder
- 2 cups baby spinach
- 1 lb lean ground turkey
- 1 can light coconut milk
- 1 tbsp tamari

HOW TO MAKE

- Preheat large saucepan over medium high heat. Add shallots and sauté for 4-5 mins. Add garlic, ginger, curry powder, salt, cook for 3 mins. Add turkey, cook for 10 mins. Add coconut milk, tamari, zucchini, spinach. Cover and simmer for 10 mins.

TURKEY COBB *Salad*

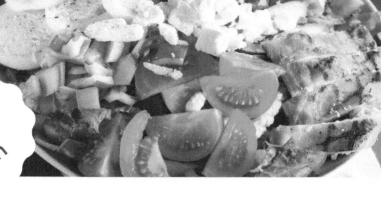

Lunch

INGREDIENTS

For 4 servings

- 4 boiled eggs, *peeled*
- 1½ cup cherry tomatoes
- 1 cup cooked turkey, *shredded*
- 5 cups lettuce, *chopped*
- ½ cup feta cheese, *reduced fat*
- ½ cup red onion, *chopped*
- 4 tbsp ranch dressing

HOW TO MAKE

- Divide lettuce between 4 bowls. Starting with eggs, arrange the remaining ingredients in rows on the lettuce.
- Drizzle 2 tbsp of ranch dressing.

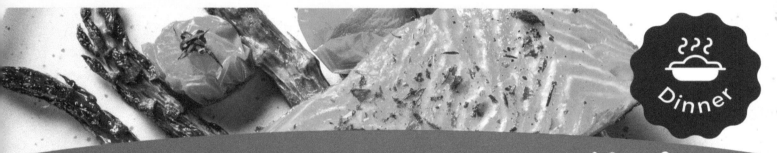

Dinner

SALMON & ASPARAGUS *Bake*

INGREDIENTS

For 4 servings

- 1 onion, *thinly sliced*
- 4 (4-oz) salmon fillets
- ½ cup cherry tomatoes
- 1 lb asparagus
- ¼ cup dijon mustard
- 1 tbsp cup olive oil
- 3 tsp Monk fruit sweetener

HOW TO MAKE

- Place onion and tomatoes in the middle of the baking sheet. Place the salmon fillets on top and place the asparagus around.
- In a small bowl, whisk together mustard, olive oil, sweetener. Spread mixture on top of the salmon fillets.
- Preheat oven to 400°F. Bake 20 mins.

SWEET POTATO *Soup*

Lunch

INGREDIENTS

For 4 servings

- 1 tbsp olive oil
- 1 onion, *roughly chopped*
- 2 large carrots, *roughly chopped*
- 1½ in ginger, *finely chopped*
- 10 oz sweet potatoes
- 2 cups vegetable stock

HOW TO MAKE

- Heat the oil in a saucepan. Add the onion, carrots, ginger, fry for 5 mins. Add sweet potatoes, stock.
- Simmer with the lid on for 15 mins. Blend the soup.

CHICKEN BROWN RICE *Pasta*

Dinner

INGREDIENTS

For 4 servings

- 1 lb chicken breast
- 1 cup mushrooms, *sliced*
- 1 cup cherry tomatoes
- 1 large zucchini, *chopped*
- 3 tbsp basil leaves
- 2 cups brown rice pasta, *uncooked*
- 2 tbsp tamari
- ½ cup fat-free greek yogurt

HOW TO MAKE

- Bring a pot of water to the boil, add pasta. Cook until al dente.
- Heat up olive oil in a skillet. Add chicken, mushrooms, zucchini.
- When the chicken is cooked through, add halved tomatoes, tamari and heat through.
- Take the heat off, add the pasta, greek yogurt and stir to combine.
- Season with fresh basil leaves.

RED LENTIL Soup

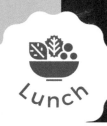

Lunch

INGREDIENTS

For 4 servings

- 1 tsp cumin seeds
- 1 tbsp olive oil
- 1 red onion, *chopped*
- 1 cup red lentils
- 4 cups vegetable stock
- 1 can tomatoes
- 1 can chickpeas

HOW TO MAKE

- Heat a large saucepan, add olive oil, cumin, onion, saute for 5 mins. Add lentils, stock, tomatoes, chickpeas, salt to taste. Simmer for 20 mins.
- Blend the soup

Dinner

LEMON TILAPIA *with Mushrooms*

INGREDIENTS

For 4 servings

- 2 tbsp olive oil
- ½ lb mushrooms, *sliced*
- ¾ tsp lemon-pepper seasoning
- 3 garlic cloves, *minced*
- 4 (6 oz) tilapia fillets
- ⅛ tsp cayenne pepper
- 1 tomato, *chopped*
- 3 green onions, *sliced*

HOW TO MAKE

- In a skillet, heat oil medium heat. Add mushrooms, ¼ tsp lemon-pepper seasoning, cook and stir 3-5 mins. Add garlic, cook 30 seconds longer.
- Place fillets over mushrooms, sprinkle with cayenne and remaining lemon pepper. Cook, covered, 7 mins. Top with tomato and green onions.

EDAMAME *Stir-Fry*

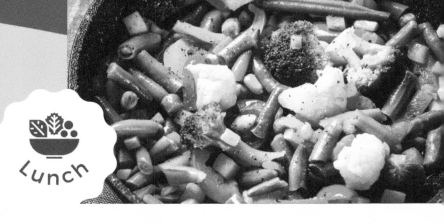

Lunch

INGREDIENTS
For 4 servings

- 14 oz shelled edamame
- 1 cup cauliflower, *chopped*
- 1 cup bell peppers, *diced*
- 4 cloves garlic, *chopped*
- 1 cup broccoli, *chopped*
- 1 cup green beans
- 2 tsp olive oil

HOW TO MAKE

- Heat oil in a pan. Sauté garlic a min. Add cauliflower, bell peppers, salt, edamame, broccoli, beans. Cover, cook until the vegetables are softened.

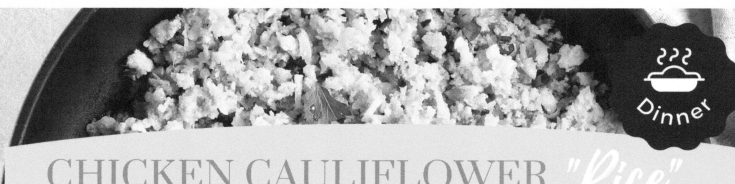

Dinner

CHICKEN CAULIFLOWER *"Rice"*

INGREDIENTS
For 4 servings

- 1 large head cauliflower
- 1 lb chicken breasts
- ½ tsp pepper
- 1 tbsp olive oil
- 1 bell pepper, *chopped*
- 1 small onion, *chopped*
- 1 garlic clove, *minced*
- ½ cup tomato juice
- ¼ cup cilantro, *chopped*

HOW TO MAKE

- Cut and pulse cauliflower in a food processor until it resembles rice.
- In a large skillet, saute chicken (cut into cubes) with salt to taste and pepper about 5 mins. Add bell pepper, onion and garlic, cook 3 mins. Stir in tomato juice. Add cauliflower. Cover, cook 7 mins. Add cilantro.

CRAB *Cakes*

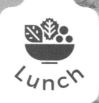

Lunch

INGREDIENTS

For 4 servings

- 1 lb lump crabmeat
- 4 small shallots, *diced*
- 4 tbsp green onions, *chopped*
- 4 tbsp fat-free greek yogurt
- 1 cup almond flour
- 2 tbsp olive oil, *for frying*
- 2 large eggs

HOW TO MAKE

- In a mixing bowl, add all of the ingredients and mix
- Form patties. In a pan add the olive oil. Fry patties for 5 mins per side.
- Serve with your favorite vegetables.

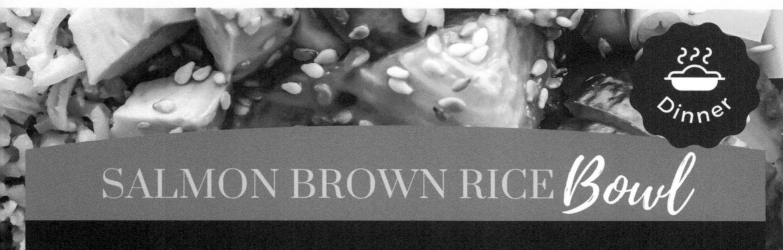

Dinner

SALMON BROWN RICE *Bowl*

INGREDIENTS

For 4 servings

- 1 cup brown rice
- 1 salmon fillet, *cubes*
- ½ cup fat-free greek yogurt
- 2 tbsp sriracha hot sauce
- ⅓ cup coconut aminos
- 3 small avocados, *sliced*
- 2 cups cucumber, *sliced*
- 6 radishes, *thinly sliced*
- 2 tbsp sesame seeds

HOW TO MAKE

- Cook brown rice.
- Heat up olive oil (2 tsp) in a skillet. Cook salmon with salt and pepper for 8 mins.
- In a bowl, whisk yogurt, sriracha and coconut aminos.
- Divide rice among 4 bowls. Top with salmon, avocado, radish, cucumber. Drizzle sauce. Sprinkle with sesame seeds.

LENTIL TOMATO *Salad*

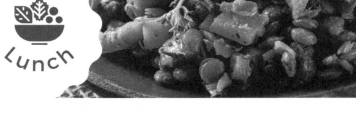

Lunch

INGREDIENTS
For 4 servings

- ¼ cup balsamic vinegar
- 1 ½ cups cherry tomatoes
- 1 can (15 oz) lentils, *drained*
- 1 red onion, *thinly sliced*
- 1 cup baby spinach, *chopped*
- ¼ cup cilantro, *chopped*

HOW TO MAKE

- Halve cherry tomatoes.
- Add all ingredients to a bowl and toss to combine. Add salt to taste and adjust vinegar.

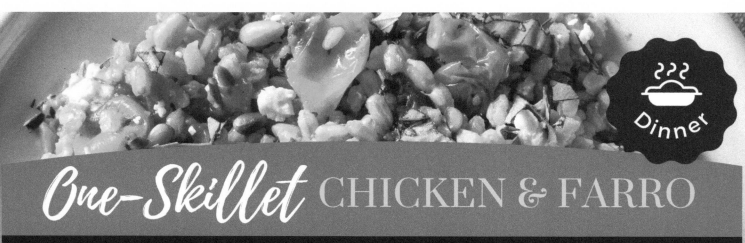

Dinner

One-Skillet CHICKEN & FARRO

INGREDIENTS
For 4 servings

- 1 lb chicken breast, *cubed*
- 1 cup onion, *diced*
- 2 cans chicken broth
- 2 cups farro
- 1 (14.5 ounce) can Italian-style diced tomatoes
- 1 cup baby spinach
- 1 tsp dried parsley
- 1 tsp basil

HOW TO MAKE

- Heat a skillet over medium heat. Cook chicken and onion 5 mins. Remove chicken.
- Pour chicken broth into skillet and bring to a boil. Stir in farro. Cover, reduce heat, cook 15 mins. Return chicken to skillet. Stir in tomatoes, spinach, basil, and parsley. Season with salt and pepper to taste. Simmer 5 mins.

ZUCCHINI *Muffins*

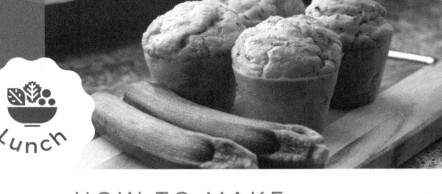

Lunch

INGREDIENTS
For 4 servings

- 3 eggs
- 1 cup wholemeal flour
- 2 cups zucchini, *grated*
- ½ cup low fat cheese, *grated*
- 1 can corn kernels, *drained*
- 1 can kidney beans, *drained*
- ¼ cup olive oil

HOW TO MAKE

- Preheat oven to 360°F.
- Whisk eggs and flour together. Add all remain ingredients. Mix.
- Divide mixture among muffin cups. Bake for 20 mins.

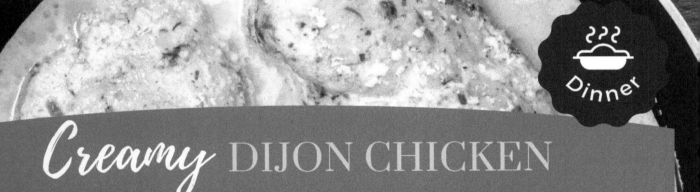

Creamy DIJON CHICKEN

Dinner

INGREDIENTS
For 4 servings

- ½ cup *nonfat* half-and-half cream
- ¼ cup dijon mustard
- 4 chicken breast halves
- 2 tsp olive oil
- 1 onion, *thinly sliced*
- 1 tsp dried thyme

HOW TO MAKE

- Whisk together cream and mustard. Sprinkle chicken with salt and pepper to taste.
- Heat oil in a large skillet. Brown chicken on both sides. Reduce heat to medium. Add onion and cream mixture, bring to a boil. Reduce heat and cook 10 mins. Sprinkle with thyme.

BROCCOLI
Fritters

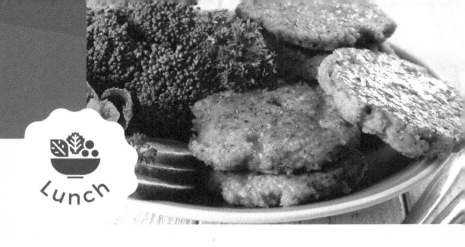

INGREDIENTS
For 4 servings

- 1 lb broccoli rice
- 10 oz hummus
- 2 small eggs
- ⅔ cup wholemeal breadcrumbs
- ½ tsp garlic powder
- ⅓ tsp salt

Lunch

HOW TO MAKE

- Thoroughly combine broccoli rice, hummus, eggs, crumbs, salt, garlic powder. Shape into fritters.
- Fry the fritters 7 mins per side.

Dinner

Creamy LENTIL CURRY

INGREDIENTS
For 4 servings

- 1 cup red lentils
- 1 (28 oz) can diced fire-roasted tomatoes
- 1 (13.5 oz) can light coconut milk
- 1 tbsp curry powder
- 1 (13.5 oz) can chickpeas, drained
- 1 cup spinach

HOW TO MAKE

- Add red lentils, coconut milk, tomatoes, curry powder, salt to taste to a saucepan. Bring to a simmer of medium-high heat for 10 mins.
- Stir in spinach and chickpeas. Simmer for 10 mins. Add salt to taste.
- Serve alone or spooned over brown rice.

KALE & QUINOA *Salad*

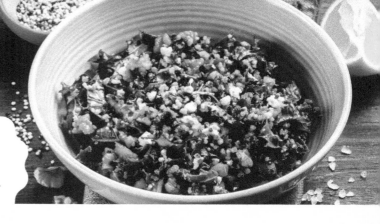

INGREDIENTS

For 4 servings

Lunch

- 2 tbsp olive oil
- 1 cup quinoa
- 1 cup kale, *roughly chopped*
- 1 cup sun-dried tomatoes
- 1 can chickpeas, *drained*
- ⅓ cup walnuts, *chopped*
- 1 tbsp lemon juice

HOW TO MAKE

- Cook quinoa according to instructions on package.
- Massage the kale. Combine all ingredient, add salt to taste. Drizzle with oil, mix once more.

VEGGIE & TOFU *Stir-Fry*

Dinner

INGREDIENTS

For 4 servings

- 18 oz extra-firm tofu
- 2 cups broccoli, *chopped*
- 1 carrot, *sliced into sticks*
- 1 tsp fresh ginger, *minced*
- 2 tbsp apple cider vinegar
  2 tbsp tahini
- 1 tsp sriracha
- ¼ cup tamari
- 1 tbsp olive oil

HOW TO MAKE

- Add oil, tofu (cut into cubes) to a skillet and cook for about 2 mins, set aside.
- Mix together sriracha, vinegar, tahini, tamari.
- Add vegetables with ¼ cup of water, cover and cook 5 mins.
- Add tofu to the veggies. Pour the sauce and cook 2 mins.

BUCKWHEAT
Bowl

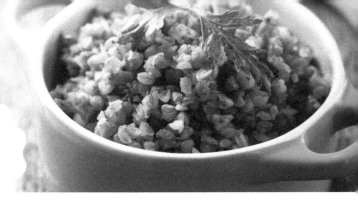

Lunch

INGREDIENTS
For 4 servings

- 1 cup buckwheat groats
- 1 cup edamame, *shelled*
- 1 sheet nori, *cut into thin strips*
- 2 tbsp sesame seeds, *toasted*
- 1 avocado, *sliced*
- 2 tbsp sriracha
- 1 cup kimchi

HOW TO MAKE

- Cook buckwheat according to instructions on package.
- Divide buckwheat among 4 bowls. Add edamame and avocado. Drizzle with sriracha, top with kimchi, nori.

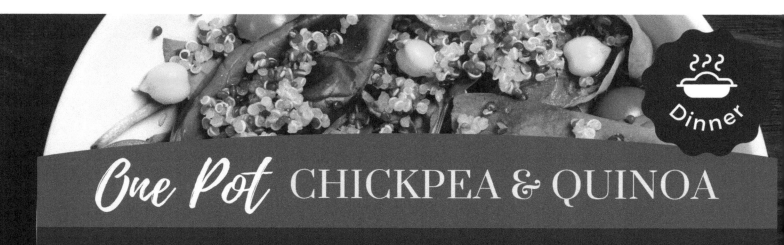

Dinner

One Pot CHICKPEA & QUINOA

INGREDIENTS
For 4 servings

- 1 tbsp olive oil
- 2 garlic cloves, *minced*
- ½ tsp dried thyme
- 1½ cup quinoa
- 1 cup green olives, *sliced*
- ½ cup sun dried tomatoes, *chopped*
- 1 cup spinach, *chopped*
- 1 can chickpeas, *drained*

HOW TO MAKE

- Cook quinoa according to instructions on package.
- Heat oil in a saucepan over medium heat. Add thyme, garlic, sauté 2 mins.
- Add quinoa, olives, tomatoes. Cook 15 seconds. Stir in spinach and chickpeas. Let sit for a 1 min. Season with salt and pepper to taste.

QUINOA *Bake*

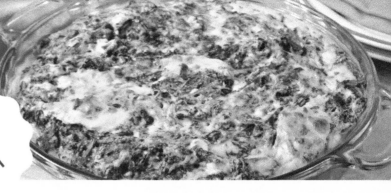

Lunch

INGREDIENTS
For 4 servings

- 1 cup quinoa
- ½ cup low fat cheese, *grated*
- 2 cups baby spinach
- ½ cup almond milk
- 1 large egg
- 1 olive oil

HOW TO MAKE

- Cook quinoa according to instructions on package.
- Whisk milk, egg, salt in a bowl.
- Add mixture, spinach, cheese to quinoa, stir. Bake 15 mins at 375°F.

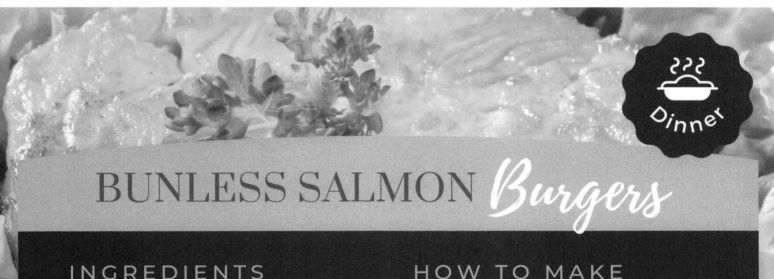

Dinner

BUNLESS SALMON *Burgers*

INGREDIENTS
For 4 servings

- 1 lb salmon fillet
- 1 cup wholemeal breadcrumbs
- 2 eggs
- ¼ cup fat-free greek yogurt
- 1 tbsp lemon juice
- 1 tsp mustard
- 2 cups lettuce
- 1 tsp olive oil

HOW TO MAKE

- Chop the salmon fillet into small pieces and transfer it into a bowl, add salt to taste.
- Stir in the rest of ingredients.
- Heat a little oil in a large non-stick grill pan over medium heat. Divide the mixture into 4 and form neat patties. Fry the patties 4 mins on each side. Serve with lettuce.

CHICKEN SLAW *Tacos*

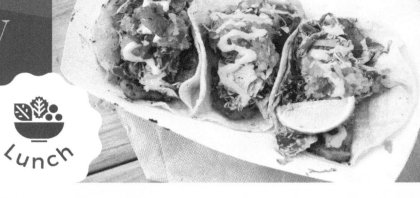

Lunch

INGREDIENTS
For 4 servings

- 1 tbsp cider vinegar
- ⅓ cup fat-free greek yogurt
- 2 cups red cabbage, *shredded*
- 2 cups cooked chicken breast, *shredded*
- 3 tbsp light barbecue sauce
- 8 corn tortillas

HOW TO MAKE

- Combine yogurt, vinegar, salt in a large bowl. Add cabbage, toss.
- Combine chicken, barbecue sauce.
- Heat tortillas. Fill each tortilla with chicken and slaw.

Dinner

CHICKEN VEGGIE *Stir-Fry*

INGREDIENTS
For 4 servings

- 2 tbsp coconut aminos
- ¾ cup chicken broth
- 2 ½ cups broccoli, *chopped*
- 1 lb chicken breasts
- 2 tbsp olive oil
- 1 ½ cups carrots, *sliced*
- 1 small yellow onion
- 1 bell pepper, *sliced*
- 1 cup peas

HOW TO MAKE

- Heat oil in a skillet over medium-high heat. Add chicken (cut into pieces). Cook 6 mins.
- Add in carrots, onions, broccoli, bell pepper, peas, saute 10 mins. Pour coconut aminos and chicken broth, saute for another 1-2 mins. tossing constantly.

BUCKWHEAT *Salad*

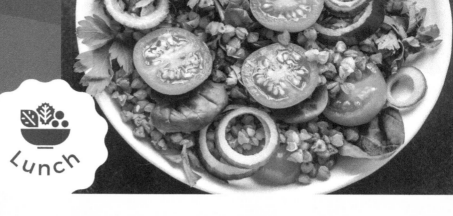

Lunch

INGREDIENTS

For 4 servings

- 1 cup buckwheat groats
- ½ cup red onion, *diced*
- 2 cups cherry tomatoes
- 1 cup pitted kalamata olives
- 1 cup baby spinach
- 2 bell peppers, sliced
- 2 tbsp olive oil

HOW TO MAKE

- Cook buckwheat according to instructions on package.
- Combine cooled groats with tomato, spinach, olives, and bell pepper in a salad bowl. Add olive oil, salt to taste.

CREAMY TUNA & PASTA *Bake*

Dinner

INGREDIENTS

For 4 servings

- 14 oz wholemeal pasta
- 1 can (12 oz) tuna, *drained*
- 1 cup spinach
- 1 can corn kernels, *drained*
- ½ cup wholemeal breadcrumbs
- 1 cup tomato sauce
- ⅓ cup reduced fat mozzarella cheese, *grated*

HOW TO MAKE

- Warm the oven to 350°F.
- Cook the pasta "al dente".
- Add the spinach for 1 min and allow to wilt.
- Drain and transfer to a baking dish. Mix in the tuna, corn and tomato sauce
- Top with mozzarella and breadcrumbs.
- Bake for 15 mins.

WHITE BEAN *Patties*

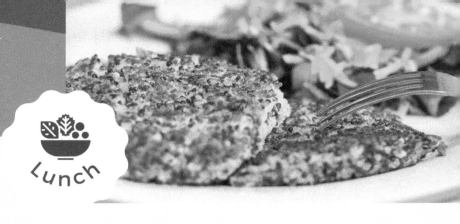

INGREDIENTS
For 4 servings

Lunch

- 2 tbsp olive oil
- 1 can (15 oz) white beans
- 4 slices wholemeal bread
- 2 tbsp nutritional yeast
- ½ tsp onion powder
- ½ tsp garlic salt
- ½ tsp of cumin

HOW TO MAKE

- In a food processor, place all ingredients and process until well incorporated. Form patties.
- Heat oil in a skillet. Cook patties until lightly brown each side.

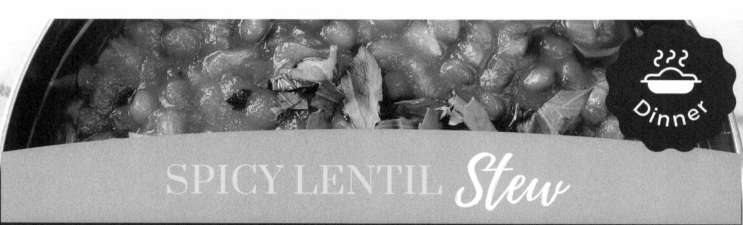

SPICY LENTIL *Stew*

Dinner

INGREDIENTS
For 4 servings

- 1 tbsp olive oil
- 1 large carrot, *diced*
- 2 celery sticks, *diced*
- 2 sweet potatoes, *diced*
- 1 garlic clove, *crushed*
- 3 tomatoes, *chopped*
- 2 ½ cups vegetable stock
- 4 tbsp fat-free greek yogurt
- 1 cup red lentils

HOW TO MAKE

- Heat the oil in a saucepan over a medium-high heat. Add the carrot, celery, garlic and potatoes, cook 5 mins.
- Stir in the tomatoes and lentils. Add the vegetable stock, salt to taste and simmer for 20 mins.
- Serve with yogurt.

Thai CAULIFLOWER

Lunch

INGREDIENTS
For 4 servings

- 1 big head cauliflower, *cut into florets*
- 2 tsp thai red curry paste
- ½ cup light coconut milk
- 1 can chickpeas, *drained*
- 1 tbsp olive oil

HOW TO MAKE

- Heat oven to 400°F. Bake (20 mins) chickpeas and cauliflower with oil.
- Combine curry paste with milk in a saucepan. Simmer 2 mins. Pour it over cauliflower and chickpeas.

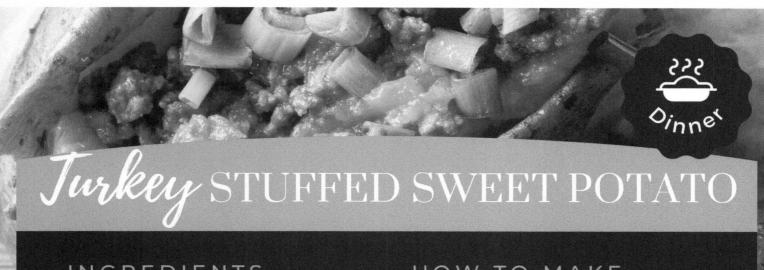

Dinner

Turkey STUFFED SWEET POTATO

INGREDIENTS
For 4 servings

- 1 green onion, *chopped*
- 4 medium sweet potatoes
- 1 lb ground turkey
- 1 can (9 oz) black beans, *drained*
- 1 cup corn kernels
- 1 tbsp taco seasoning
- ¼ cup fat-free greek yogurt
- 1 tbsp olive oil

HOW TO MAKE

- Wash potatoes thoroughly, pierce with a fork. Microwave 5 min, turning halfway.
- Cut potatoes in half and fluff their centers with a fork.
- Heat the oil in a large skillet. Add turkey, cook 10 mins. Add beans, corn, taco seasoning and mix. Spoon mixture into sweet potato, serve with yogurt.

Baked
TEMPEH

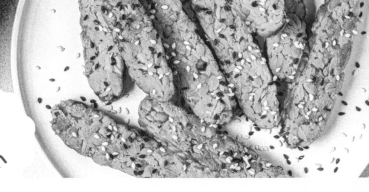

Lunch

INGREDIENTS
For 4 servings

- 16 oz block tempeh
- 2 tbsp tamari
- 2 tbsp nutritional yeast
- 1 tbsp sesame seeds
- 2 cups raw vegetables, *to serve*

HOW TO MAKE

- Cut the tempeh into cubes. Drizzle the tamari, then stir well. Sprinkle the nutritional yeast and mix again.
- Preheat the oven to 400°F.
- Bake 20 mins. Serve with veggies.

Dinner

QUINOA & SHRIMP *Stir Fry*

INGREDIENTS
For 4 servings

- 2 tbsp olive oil
- 1 onion, *finely chopped*
- 1 clove garlic minced
- ½ tsp chili powder
- 2 cups dry quinoa
- 1 lb shrimp, *peeled*
- ½ tsp chili powder
- ½ cup parsley, *chopped*
- Juice of one lemon

HOW TO MAKE

- Cook quinoa according to instructions on package.
- Heat the olive oil in a skillet. Add the onion, garlic, cook 3 mins. Add the shrimp, chili powder, salt. Sauté until no longer translucent.
- Mix the quinoa and shrimp, drizzle with lemon juice, sprinkle with parsley.

CAULIFLOWER
Muffins

Lunch

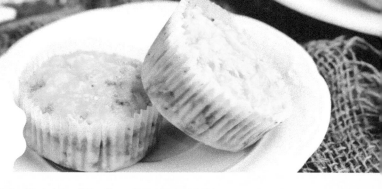

INGREDIENTS
For 4 servings

- 4 cups cauliflower rice
- ½ cup onion, *diced*
- 1½ cups low fat cheese, *shredded*
- 1 tsp Italian seasoning
- 2 eggs

HOW TO MAKE

- Preheat oven to 350°F.
- Mix all ingredients in a large bowl. Scoop mixture into muffin cups.
- Bake for 25 mins or until firm and starting to brown.

Dinner

Almond CRUSTED FISH

INGREDIENTS
For 4 servings

- 1 egg
- 1 lb fish fillets
- ½ cup sliced almonds
- 1 cup wholemeal breadcrumbs
- 3 tbsp almond milk
- ¼ tsp chili powder
- 2 tbsp olive oil

HOW TO MAKE

- Prepare one bowl with egg and milk, and one bowl with breadcrumbs, chopped almonds, salt. Dip each fillet, one at a time into egg mixture then into almond mixture.
- Preheat oven to 450 °F. Bake in oven with oil for 6 mins per side, flipping halfway.

BLACK BEAN *Soup*

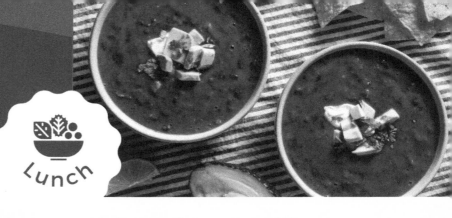

Lunch

INGREDIENTS

For 4 servings

- 1 tbsp olive oil
- 1 medium onion, *chopped*
- 1 tsp ground cumin
- 2 cloves garlic
- 2 cans (14 oz) black beans
- 2 cups vegetable broth
- ½ cup avocado, *cubes*

HOW TO MAKE

- Saute onion in olive oil. Add cumin, garlic and cook 30 seconds. Add black beans and vegetable broth. Bring to a simmer. Blend the ingredients. Serve with avocado.

Dinner

Spicy COCONUT SHRIMP

INGREDIENTS

For 4 servings

- 2 tbsp olive oil
- 1 cup onion, *chopped*
- 1 tbsp garlic, *minced*
- 2 tsp ginger, *minced*
- ⅛ tsp turmeric
- 1 cup canned tomato
- 1 cup light coconut milk
- 1 ½ lbs large shrimp, *peeled*
- ¾ cup broccoli, *chopped*

HOW TO MAKE

- Heat oil in skillet. Add onions and stir for 3 mins. Add garlic and ginger, cook 2 mins. Add spices and cook 1 min. Add tomatoes, broccoli, cook 2 mins. Add coconut milk, ½ cup water, and salt. Simmer until thickened 5-10 mins. Add shrimp, simmer 5 mins.

TUNA STUFFED *Avocado*

Lunch

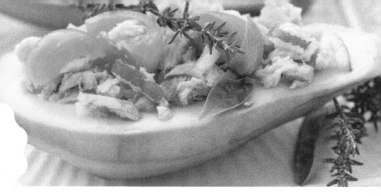

INGREDIENTS
For 4 servings

- 4 avocados, *halved*
- 4 cans (4.5 oz) tuna, *drained*
- ½ cup red onion, *diced*
- ½ cup cherry tomatoes, *halved*
- 1 tbsp lime juice

HOW TO MAKE

- Scoop out some of the avocado.
- Add the tuna, onion to the bowl. Pour lime juice. Stir together.
- Scoop the tuna into the avocado. Add tomatoes.

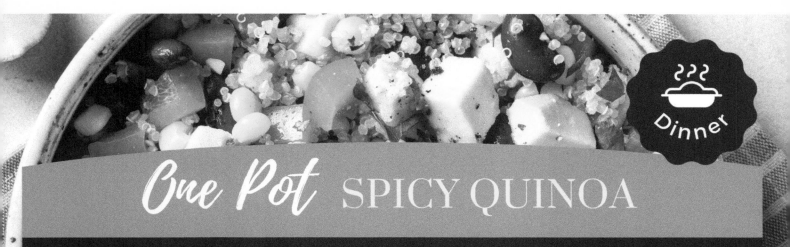

Dinner

One Pot SPICY QUINOA

INGREDIENTS
For 4 servings

- 1 onion, *sliced*
- 4 tbsp curry paste
- 4 cups almond milk
- 1½ cups frozen mixed vegetable
- 2 cups dry quinoa
- Avocado, *to serve*
- 1 can (15 oz) kidney beans

HOW TO MAKE

- Simmer the onion and the curry paste with a splash of water for 5 mins. Add the vegetables and quinoa, add salt to taste then stir in the milk. Bring to the boil, simmer gently for 10 mins until the quinoa is cooked.
- Serve with avocado, beans.

SALMON Tartare

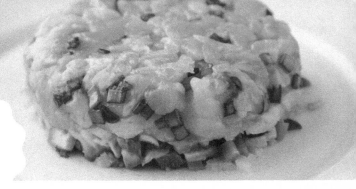

Lunch

INGREDIENTS
For 4 servings

- 1 tbsp olive oil
- 8 oz smoked salmon, *chopped*
- 2 spring onions, *chopped*
- 2 tbsp shallot, *chopped*
- 2 avocados, *chopped*

HOW TO MAKE

- Mix salmon with oil, shallots.
- Use measuring cup as a mold, and pack with the salmon mixture, top with avocado. Turn out onto plate. Garnish with spring onions.

Dinner

TOMATO TUNA Curry

INGREDIENTS
For 4 servings

- 4 tuna steaks
- 1 tsp red chili powder
- 1 tsp ginger powder
- ½ tsp turmeric powder
- 3 red dried chilies, *halved*
- 2 tomatoes, *chopped*
- 1 onion, chopped
- 1 cup fish stock
- 1 tbsp olive oil

HOW TO MAKE

- Cut the tuna into medium chunks.
- Heat oil in saucepan. Add the onion and cook 1 min. Add the turmeric, chili powder, ginger powder, tomato, cook 6 mins. Pour in the fish stock. Bring it to boil. Add the fish, chili, and cook 15 mins.

BEAN BURRITO *Bowl*

Lunch

INGREDIENTS
For 4 servings

- 2 (15oz) cans black beans
- 4 tbsp low fat cheese
- 1 can (15oz) corn kernels
- 4 tbsp tomato salsa
- 1 tsp ground cumin
- 1 tsp garlic powder
- 1½ cup brown rice

HOW TO MAKE

- Cook brown rice according to instructions.
- Drain and warm beans and corn.
- Serve rice with beans, corn, salsa, leftover chicken *(if you have)*, cheese.

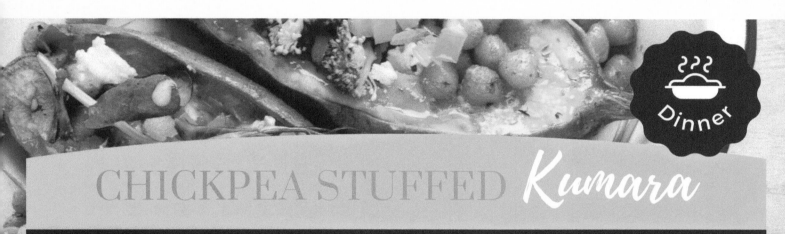

Dinner

CHICKPEA STUFFED *Kumara*

INGREDIENTS
For 4 servings

- 1 cup broccoli, *chopped*
- 1 medium bell pepper, *finely chopped*
- 4 medium kumara
- 1 can (15 oz) chickpeas, *drained*
- 1 tbsp olive oil

HOW TO MAKE

- Wash kumara thoroughly, pierce with a fork. Microwave 5 mins, turning halfway. Cut kumara in half and fluff their centers with a fork.
- Bake broccoli, bell pepper, chickpeas 15 mins at 375 °F.
- Spoon chickpeas into each kumara. Top with broccoli, bell pepper. Drizzle with oil.

BAKED SALMON *Balls*

Lunch

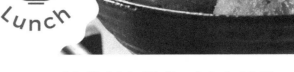

INGREDIENTS
For 4 servings

- 3 cans (6 oz) salmon
- 4 tbsp wholemeal breadcrumbs
- 2 scallion, *thinly sliced*
- 2 eggs, *lightly beaten*
- 2 tbsp fat-free greek yogurt
- 1 tbsp garlic, *minced*

HOW TO MAKE

- Preheat oven to 400°F.
- Combine all ingredients. Roll mixture into balls. Bake, flipping once, about 20 mins.

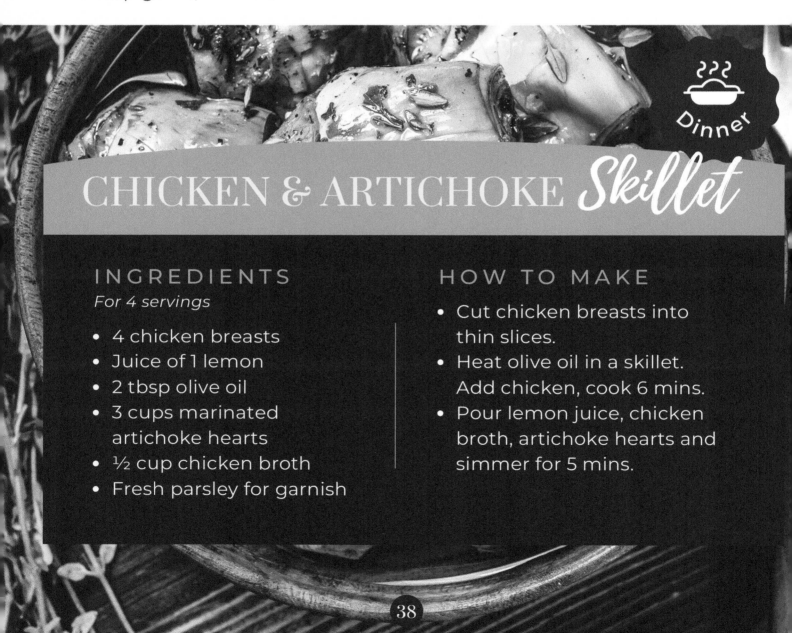

CHICKEN & ARTICHOKE *Skillet*

Dinner

INGREDIENTS
For 4 servings

- 4 chicken breasts
- Juice of 1 lemon
- 2 tbsp olive oil
- 3 cups marinated artichoke hearts
- ½ cup chicken broth
- Fresh parsley for garnish

HOW TO MAKE

- Cut chicken breasts into thin slices.
- Heat olive oil in a skillet. Add chicken, cook 6 mins.
- Pour lemon juice, chicken broth, artichoke hearts and simmer for 5 mins.

GREEK CHICKPEA *Salad*

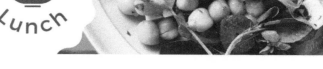

Lunch

INGREDIENTS
For 4 servings

- 1 can (15oz) chickpeas
- 2 cups cherry tomatoes
- ½ cup fresh basil
- ¼ cup onion, *slivered*
- 1 cup low fat feta cheese
- 2 tbsp olive oil
- 2 tbsp apple cider vinegar

HOW TO MAKE

- In a large bowl mix all vegetable and chickpeas.
- Drizzle with the olive oil and vinegar, season with salt to taste. Toss gently. Add feta cheese.

Dinner

CURRY TURKEY *Stir-Fry*

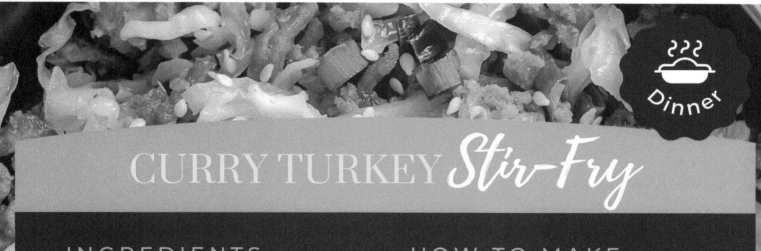

INGREDIENTS
For 4 servings

- 1 lb turkey breast strips
- 1 medium carrot, *sliced*
- 2 cups cabbage, *chopped*
- 1 cup vegetable broth
- 2 tsp curry powder
- ½ tsp ground ginger

HOW TO MAKE

- Heat oil in skillet, Add turkey, salt to taste, cook 5 mins. Stir in carrot and cabbage. Cook 2 mins.
- In small bowl, mix remaining ingredients. Stir into turkey and vegetables. Heat to boiling, reduce heat. Cover and cook until turkey is no longer pink in center.

CAULIFLOWER *Taco Bowl*

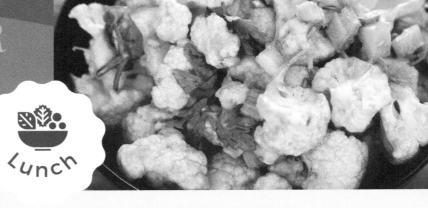

Lunch

INGREDIENTS

For 4 servings

- 6 cups cauliflower florets
- ½ cup sweet onion, *diced*
- 3 cloves garlic, *minced*
- 2 tbsp olive oil
- 1 tbsp chili powder
- 1 can (15oz) black beans

HOW TO MAKE

- Mix cauliflower, diced onion, olive oil, chili powder, and salt to taste.
- Preheat the oven to 400°F. Bake 20 mins. Serve with beans.

Dinner

COD AND ASPARAGUS *Bake*

INGREDIENTS

For 4 servings

- 4 cod fillets (4 oz each)
- 1 lb thin asparagus, trimmed
- 2 cups cherry tomatoes, halved
- 2 tbsp lemon juice
- 1 tsp grated lemon zest
- ¼ cup reduced fat cheese, grated

HOW TO MAKE

- Place cod and asparagus in baking pan brushed with oil. Add tomatoes. Dizzle fish with lemon juice and sprinkle with lemon zest, salt to taste. Top with cheese.
- Preheat oven to 400°. Bake 15 mins.

MISO CHICKEN *Stir-fry*

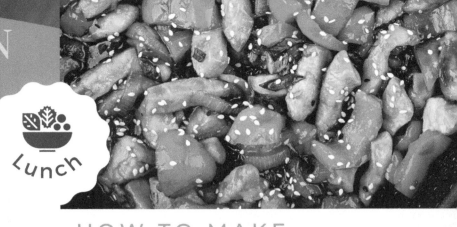

Lunch

INGREDIENTS

For 4 servings

- 3 chicken breasts, *cut into bite size pieces*
- 2 tbsp olive oil
- 2 cloves garlic, *chopped*
- 2 bell peppers, *chopped*
- 2 tbsp yellow miso paste
- 1 tbsp coconut aminos

HOW TO MAKE

- Heat the oil in skillet. Add in the chicken pieces, cook 5 mins.
- Add garlic, peppers and cook 1 min. Add miso paste, coconut aminos and mix. Cook for 1-2 mins.

PEPPER & KIDNEY BEAN *Stew*

Dinner

INGREDIENTS

For 4 servings

- 1 can (15 oz) kidney beans, *drained*
- 1 can (11 oz) corn kernels, *drained*
- 1 can (15 oz) crushed tomatoes
- 1 tbsp olive oil
- 1 red onion, *diced*
- 1 tsp smoked paprika
- ½ tsp ground cinnamon
- 2 carrots, *chopped*
- 2 cups vegetable broth

HOW TO MAKE

- Heat the oil in skillet, add the onion and cook for 1 min. Add paprika, cook for 1 min. Stir in the carrots, broth, kidney beans and canned tomatoes.
- Simmer 15 mins. Add corn and cook 2 mins.

QUINOA *Soup*

Lunch

INGREDIENTS

For 4 servings

- 2 tbsp olive oil
- 1 can (15 oz) cannellini beans
- 1 medium onion, *chopped*
- 1 large zucchini, *chopped*
- *8 cups vegetable broth*
- 2 carrots, *chopped*
- 1 cup quinoa

HOW TO MAKE

- Heat oil In a large pot. Add onion, carrot, salt to taste. Cook 5 mins.
- Add zucchini, beans, quinoa, cumin.
- Pour in broth and stir to combine.
- Bring to a boil and boil 15 mins.

Dinner

Sauteed BRUSSELS SPROUTS

INGREDIENTS

For 4 servings

- 2 tbsp olive oil
- 1 lb brussels sprouts
- 1 tbsp balsamic vinegar
- 1 tbsp english mustard
- 1 can (15 oz) lentils
- 1 tbsp olive oil
- ½ cup parsley

HOW TO MAKE

- Heat the oil in skillet, add brussels sprouts and cook 10 mins. Stir in lentils and remove from heat.
- Place brussels sprouts with lentils in a large bowl. Add balsamic vinegar, english mustard and chopped parsley, mix well to combine. Serve warm.

CASHEW THAI *Salad*

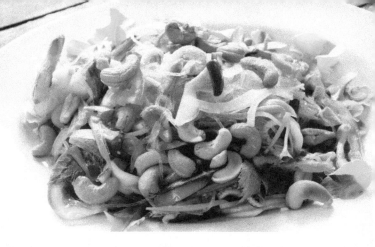

INGREDIENTS
For 4 servings

Lunch

- ¼ cup lime juice
- 1 tbsp tamari
- 2 cups lettuce
- 2 tsp olive oil
- 2 cups carrot, finely shredded
- ¼ cup onion, thinly sliced
- 1½ cups roasted cashews

HOW TO MAKE

- In a large bowl mix all vegetables and cashews.
- Drizzle with the tamari, oil and lime juice. Toss gently.

FAJITA CHICKEN *Traybake*

Dinner

INGREDIENTS
For 4 servings

- 2 tbsp olive oil
- 2 red onions, sliced
- 2 tbsp fajita spice mix
- 3 mixed peppers, *sliced*
- 1 lb mini chicken fillets
- 1 can (15 oz) black beans, *drained*
- ½ cup fat-free greek yogurt
- 2 tbsp chopped coriander

HOW TO MAKE

- Preheat the oven to 400°F.
- In a large bowl, mix fajita spice, oil, onions, peppers and chicken. Tip into the hot baking sheet. Roast in the oven for 10 mins. Stir and cook for 5 mins.
- Mix in beans, bake for 5 mins.
- Serve with the greek yogurt and coriander.

KALE BEAN
Bowl

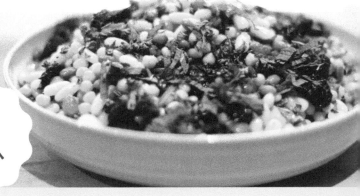

Lunch

INGREDIENTS
For 4 servings

- 1 clove garlic, *minced*
- 6 cups kale, *chopped*
- 2 cans (15oz) white beans
- ¼ cup walnuts, *chopped*
- ½ tbsp Italian seasoning
- 1 tbsp apple cider vinegar
- 1 tbsp olive oil

HOW TO MAKE

- Heat the oil in skillet, add kale and garlic. Sauté until the kale is wilted, Add bean and cook 1 min.
- Mix kale with the rest of ingredients serve warm

Dinner

LENTIL ZUCCHINI *Boats*

INGREDIENTS
For 4 servings

- 2 tbsp tamari
- 1 tbsp olive oil
- 1 medium onion, *chopped*
- 1 can (15 oz) lentils
- 4 medium zucchini
- ½ cup walnuts, *chopped*
- 1 can (15 oz) tomatoes
- ½ tsp Italian seasoning
- ½ cup low fat cheese, *grated*

HOW TO MAKE

- Cut the zucchini in half lengthwise, remove some of the flesh of the zucchini.
- Heat the oil in skillet. Fry onion, for a min. Add zucchini flesh, lentils, tamari, tomatoes, walnuts, spices. Cook 5 mins.
- Arrange lentil mixture in the zucchini boats, sprinkle with cheese, bake 10 mins at 400°F.

FISH *Tacos*

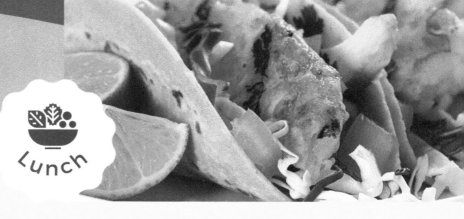

Lunch

INGREDIENTS
For 4 servings

- 1 lb fish fillets
- ½ cup fat-free greek yogurt
- 2 cups red cabbage, *shredded*
- 12 taco-sized corn tortillas
- 2 tomatoes, *thinly sliced*
- 4 radishes, *thinly sliced*
- 1 avocado, *sliced*

HOW TO MAKE

- Sprinkle the fish with salt. Add fish to the pan and cook for 2 mins. Flip fish and cook another 2 mins.
- Assemble the tacos with a few pieces of fish and other ingredients.

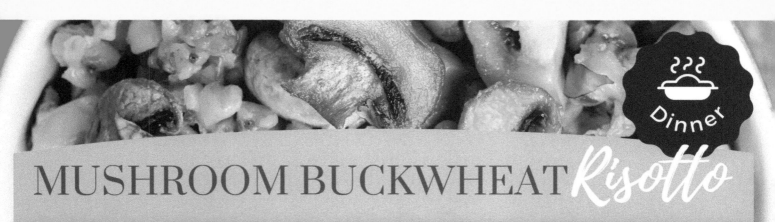

Dinner

MUSHROOM BUCKWHEAT *Risotto*

INGREDIENTS
For 4 servings

- 1½ cup buckwheat
- 16 oz mushrooms, *diced*
- 1 medium onion, *chopped*
- 1 cup green onions, *diced*
- 2 tbsp olive oil

HOW TO MAKE

- Cook buckwheat according to instructions on package.
- Heat the oil in skillet. Add onions and mushrooms cook until it becomes golden brown.
- Combine mushroom mixture with buckwheat, let it sit for about 5 mins to allow flavors to come together.

LENTIL TUNA *Salad*

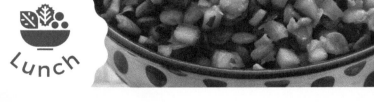

Lunch

INGREDIENTS
For 4 servings

- 1 tbsp apple cider vinegar
- 1 tsp Dijon mustard
- 2 garlic cloves, *minced*
- 2 tbsp olive oil
- 1 (15 oz) can lentils, *drained*
- 2 (6 oz) cans tuna, *drained*
- 2 bell peppers, *chopped*

HOW TO MAKE

- Whisk the vinegar, mustard, oil, garlic together.
- Add the lentils, tuna, peppers to a large bowl and toss together. Pour over the dressing and toss again.

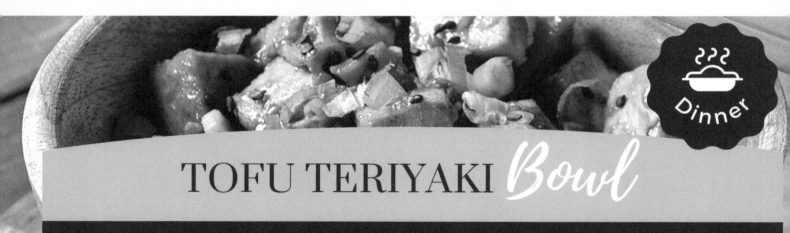

Dinner

TOFU TERIYAKI *Bowl*

INGREDIENTS
For 4 servings

- 14 oz. firm tofu, *cut in cubes*
- 1 tsp ginger, *freshly grated*
- 1 medium onion, *sliced*
- 2 spring onions, *chopped*
- 3 tsp Monk fruit sweetener
- 2 cups brown rice
- 2 tbsp olive oil
- 2 tbsp tamari

HOW TO MAKE

- Cook rice according to instructions on package.
- Heat the oil in skillet. Add tofu to the pan, fry 5 mins.
- Add the ginger, onions, tamari, sweetener. Stir-fry for 2-3 mins.
- Serve over rice with spring onions

SALMON *Rolls*

Lunch

INGREDIENTS

For 4 servings

- 8 large slices smoked salmon
- 1 cup low fat cream cheese
- 2 tbsp horseradish
- 1 tbsp lemon juice
- ½ cup cucumber sticks
- ½ cup carrot sticks

HOW TO MAKE

- Whisk cream cheese with horseradish, lemon juice.
- Spread cream cheese mixture onto salmon slices and top with cucumber and carrot sticks. Roll up.

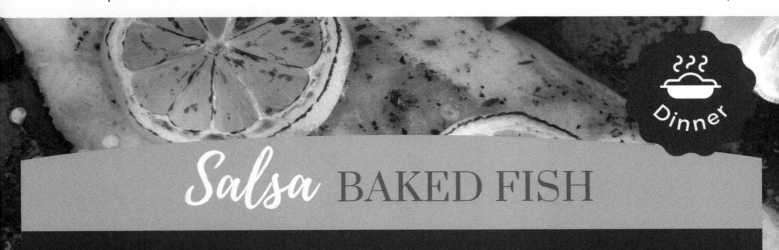

Dinner

Salsa BAKED FISH

INGREDIENTS

For 4 servings

- 1 cup barley
- 1 tbsp olive oil
- 1 lb white fish
- 1 cup salsa
- 1 small zucchini, *diced*
- 2 bell peppers
- 1 cup tomatoes, *chopped*
- 2 garlic cloves, *minced*
- ½ lemon

HOW TO MAKE

- Cook barley according to instructions on package.
- Place all vegetables into a bowl, drizzle in enough olive oil, salt and pepper to taste.
- Generously top the filets with the salsa, add in a few lemon wedges. Place vegetables around. Bake 15 mins at 400°F.
- Serve with barley.

AVOCADO EGG
Sandwiches

Lunch

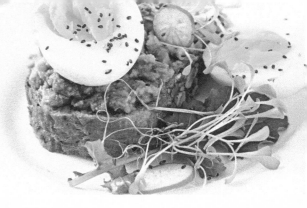

INGREDIENTS
For 4 servings

- Juice 1 lime
- 8 slices rye bread
- 4 boiled eggs
- 2 ripe avocados
- 4 tsp hot sriracha
- Handful cress, to serve

HOW TO MAKE

- Spread the avocado on bread. Cut the eggs in half and place on top of the avocado.
- Drizzle some chilli sauce over the eggs, top with cress.

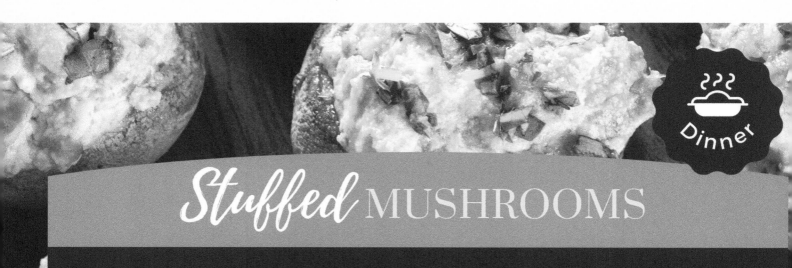

Dinner

Stuffed MUSHROOMS

INGREDIENTS
For 4 servings

- 2 cups quinoa
- ½ cup wholemeal breadcrumbs
- ½ cup low fat cheese, *grated*
- 2 garlic cloves, *minced*
- 2 tbsp parsley, *chopped*
- 1 tbsp olive oil
- 12 large portobello mushroom caps

HOW TO MAKE

- Cook quinoa according to instructions on package.
- Stir the breadcrumbs, cheese, garlic, parsley, salt to taste, olive oil together.
- Spoon the filling into the mushroom and arrange on the baking sheet.
- Bake 25 mins at 400°F.
- Serve with quinoa.

BULGUR
Bean Salad

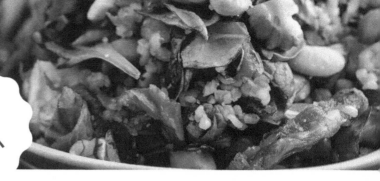

Lunch

INGREDIENTS
For 4 servings

- 1 cup bulgur
- 1 cup shelled edamame
- 1 cup sun-dried tomatoes
- 1 cup basil, *chopped*
- ½ cup green onions, *chopped*
- ¼ cup lemon juice
- 2 tbsp olive oil

HOW TO MAKE

- Cook bulgur according to instructions on package.
- Cook edamame in boiling water 3 mins. Drain.
- Add all ingredient to bulgur, mix.

SWEET POTATO & BEAN *Skillet*

Dinner

INGREDIENTS
For 4 servings

- 1 tbsp olive oil
- 2 cups sweet potato, *diced*
- 1 ½ tsp chili powder
- 1 tsp ground cumin
- 1 tsp dried oregano
- ½ tsp smoked paprika
- 4 oz green chiles, *diced*
- ½ cup salsa
- 1 (15 oz) can black beans

HOW TO MAKE

- Heat oil in a skillet. Add potatoes, salt to taste, sauté over medium heat 10 mins. Add 4 tbsp of water and cover it with a lid. Let the sweet potatoes steam 4 mins.
- Add remain ingredients. Stir everything together. Cover the skillet with lid. Cook for another 4 mins.

CREAMY CARROT *Bean Soup*

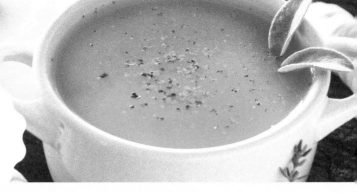

Lunch

INGREDIENTS
For 4 servings

- 2 tbsp olive oil
- 1 clove garlic, *minced*
- 1 red onion, *diced*
- 4 cups vegetable stock
- 2 cups carrots, *cut into coins*
- 1 (15 oz) can cannellini beans

HOW TO MAKE

- Add the oil to a pot. Add the garlic, onion and cook 2 mins.
- Add the vegetable stock, carrots, beans (drained). Cook 15 mins.
- Puree with blender, add salt to taste

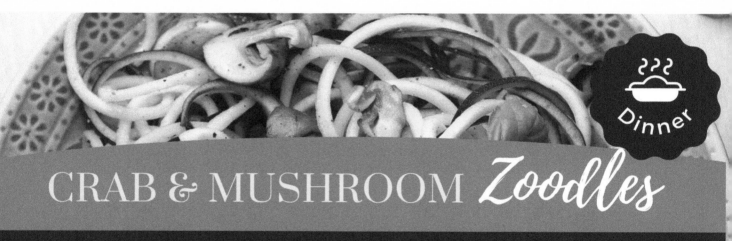

Dinner

CRAB & MUSHROOM *Zoodles*

INGREDIENTS
For 4 servings

- 2 cups jumbo lump crab meat
- 1 cup mushrooms, *chopped*
- 4 zucchinis, *peeled, noodles trimmed*
- 1 garlic clove, *minced*
- 2 tsp olive oil
- 1 avocado
- 1 lime juiced

HOW TO MAKE

- Heat olive oil in a skillet. Add the mushrooms, salt to taste. Cook 7 mins.
- Blend avocado, garlic, lime juice in a blender until creamy.
- Place the zucchini noodles into a bowl, add avocado sauce, toss until combined. Add the crab, mushrooms and toss again.

HUMMUS
Bowl

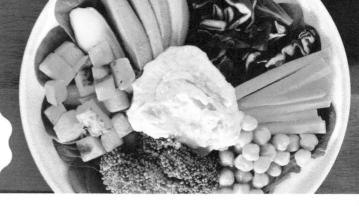

Lunch

INGREDIENTS
For 4 servings

- 2 avocados, *sliced*
- 2 cups carrot sticks
- 2 cups red cabbage, *shredded*
- 1 tbsp lemon juice
- 2 tbsp tahini
- 2 garlic cloves
- 1 tbsp olive oil

HOW TO MAKE

- Bend until creamy: lemon juice, garlic, chickpeas, oil, tahini, salt.
- Spoon the hummus onto a bowl.
- Assemble the remaining ingredients on top of the hummus.

Dinner

Shrimp BRUSSELS SPROUTS

INGREDIENTS
For 4 servings

- 1 tbsp apple cider vinegar
- 1 tbsp tamari
- 2 tsp ginger, *grated*
- 1 lb shrimp, *peeled*
- 2 tbsp olive oil
- 1 lb brussels sprouts, *trimmed*
- 3 cloves garlic, *thinly sliced*
- 1 red onion, *sliced*

HOW TO MAKE

- Whisk together vinegar, tamari and ginger. Add shrimp and toss to combine. Let it sit 10 mins.
- Preheat oven to 400°F. Place the shrimp on baking sheet in the center.
- Surround the shrimp with brussels sprouts, onion. Bake for 10-15 mins.

BREAKFASTS

OATMEAL PANCAKES

For 4 servings

- 2⅓ cups oat flour
- 3 tbsp flaxseed meal
- 2 tsp baking powder
- 2 cups almond milk
- 1 tsp olive oil

Blend all ingredient, salt to taste in blender to make batter. In a skillet set over medium heat, brush some oil. Pour batter, fry until you see bubbles form. Then flip and fry on the other side until golden brown.

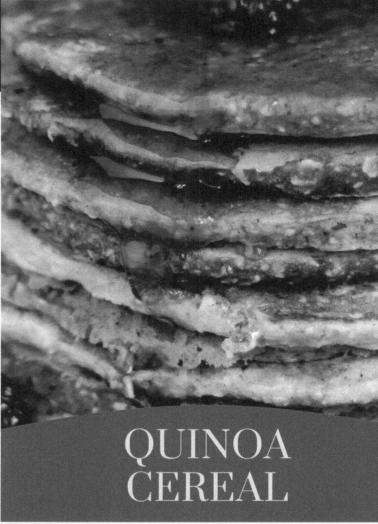

QUINOA CEREAL

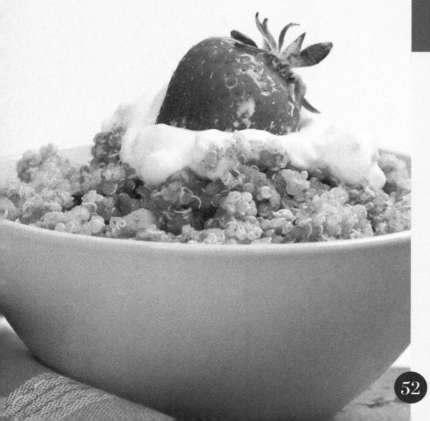

For 4 servings

- 4 cups almond milk
- 2 cups rinsed quinoa
- 2 tsp Monk fruit sweetener
- Pinch of ground cinnamon
- ½ cup fat-free greek yogurt
- Fresh berries

Bring milk and quinoa to a boil in saucepan. Simmer, covered, about 14 mins. Remove from heat and stir in sweetener, cinnamon. Top with yogurt and berries.

BREAKFASTS

SPINACH EGG MUFFINS

For 4 servings

- ½ cup dried tomatoes, *sliced*
- 1 cup spinach, *finely diced*
- ½ onion, *finely diced*
- 8 large eggs
- ¼ cup almond milk
- ⅓ cup low fat feta cheese crumbles

Preheat oven to 400°F. Process milk, eggs, spinach, salt and pepper to taste in food processor. Pour the egg mixture into the muffin tin. Add in tomatoes, onions. Bake 20 mins.

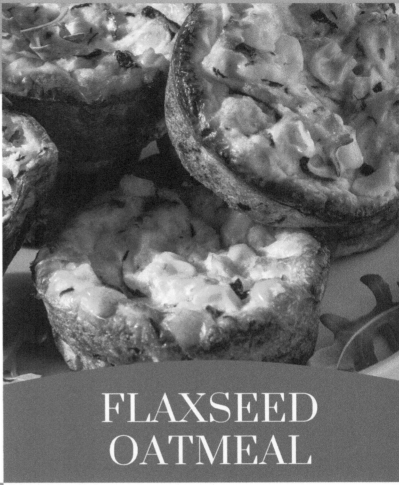

FLAXSEED OATMEAL

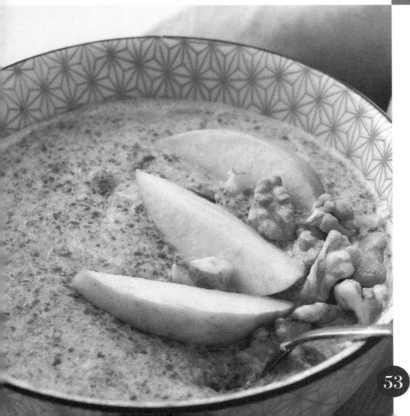

For 4 servings

- 2 cups almond milk
- 2 cup rolled oats
- 4 tbsp walnuts, *chopped*
- 2 tsp Monk fruit sweetener
- 1 cup fresh blueberries
- 4 tbsp flaxseed meal
- 2 apples

In a saucepan bring milk and water (1 ½ cup) to a boil. Reduce the heat to medium-low and stir in oats, flaxseed, and salt. Cook for 6-7 mins, uncovered. Serve with apple and walnuts.

BREAKFASTS

BUCKWHEAT PANCAKES

For 4 servings

- 1 cup buckwheat flour
- 2 tsp Monk fruit sweetener
- 2 tsp baking soda
- ⅛ tsp salt
- 1 ¼ cups almond milk
- 2 eggs

Blend all ingredient in blender to make batter. In a skillet set over medium heat, brush some oil. Pour batter, fry until you see bubbles form. Flip and fry on the other side until golden brown.

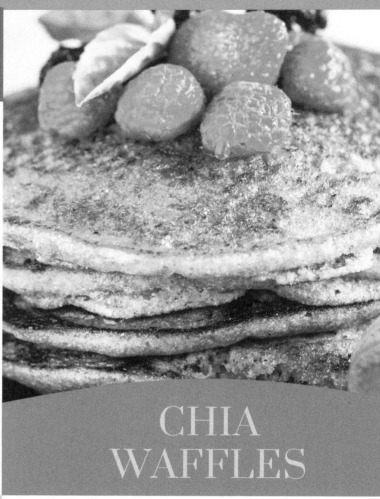

CHIA WAFFLES

For 4 servings

- 1 ¾ cups almond milk
- ½ cup applesauce
- 1 egg, *beaten*
- 2 tsp chia seeds
- ½ cup whole wheat flour
- 1 ¼ cups rolled oats
- ¼ cup flaxseed meal
- 4 tsp baking powder
- 1 tbsp Monk fruit sweetener

Blend all ingredient in blender. Scoop ½ cup batter into the preheated waffle iron and cook about 5 mins per waffle.

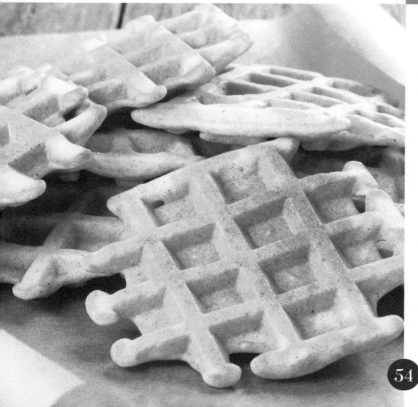

Air Fryer Meals

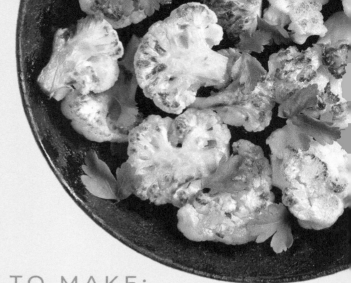

CRISPY CAULIFLOWER

INGREDIENTS:

For 4 servings

- 1 medium head of cauliflower
- 2 tbsp olive oil
- 1 tsp garlic powder
- ½ tsp smoked paprika
- ½ tsp turmeric powder

HOW TO MAKE:

Cut the cauliflower into florets. In a large bowl, add the florets, spices, salt and pepper to taste, olive oil and toss the florets so the spices are evenly coated.
Preheat Air fryer at 380°F for 5 mins. Place cauliflower in a single layer in Air fryer basket. Cook 10 mins.

ZUCCHINI FRIES

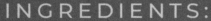

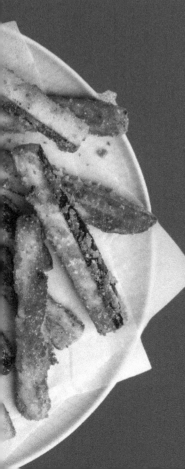

INGREDIENTS:

For 4 servings

- 2 zucchinis cut into fries
- ⅔ cup almond flour
- ¼ cup low fat cheese
- 1 tsp smoked paprika
- Olive oil spray

HOW TO MAKE:

- Combine almond flour, cheese, paprika, salt to taste in a bowl.
- Spray zucchini with olive oil.
- Dip zucchini fries into the cheese mixture.
- Preheat Air fryer at 400°F for 5 mins. Place fries in a single layer. Cook 7-10 mins.

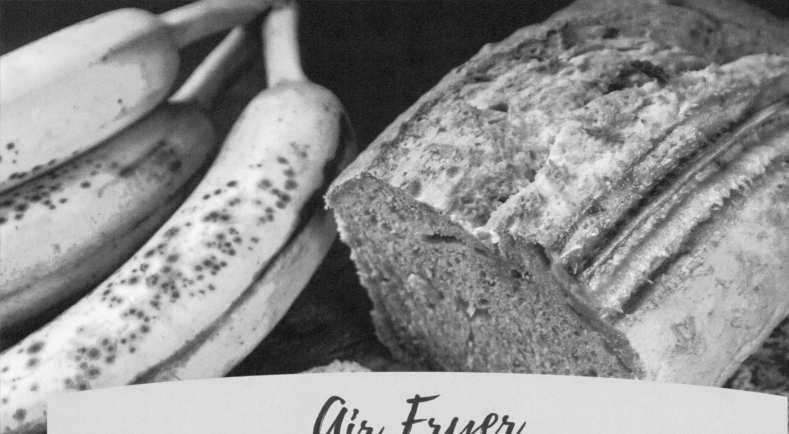

Air Fryer
BANANA BREAD

INGREDIENTS
For 4 servings

- 1 ⅓ cups whole wheat flour
- ½ cups almond milk
- 1 tsp baking powder
- 1 tsp baking soda
- 1 tsp cinnamon
- ½ cup of olive oil
- 6 overripe bananas

HOW TO MAKE

- Mix together all of the ingredients in a mixer.
- Then spray your pan with non-stick cooking spray
- Cook in the Air Fryer at 400°F for 20-25 mins.

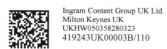

Ingram Content Group UK Ltd.
Milton Keynes UK
UKHW050358280323
419243UK00003B/110

9 798987 352045